Let's

heal together

workbook

● ● ●

THE BREAKUP EDITION

by: Cordelia
kovalic, j.d.

a note about legal and publishing info

This author's intention in writing this workbook is to provide helpful information regarding the subject matter covered. The author is not engaged in rendering psychological, financial, legal, or other professional services to the reader. If expert assistance is needed, the reader should seek the services of a competent professional.

The reader should not use this workbook to diagnose or treat any medical condition. For diagnosis or treatment of any medical problem, consult the appropriate provider.

Written by Calli Cordelia Kovalic

Cover and page designs by Kerrie Legend

Edited by Kasi Alexander

ISBN (paperback): 978-1-7358566-0-5
ISBN (ebook): 978-1-7358566-1-2

This workbook is dedicated to all those

who feel left reeling after a breakup or divorce.

who feel rejected, brokenhearted, or unsure of who they are.

May you find peace.
you are stronger than
you will ever know.

xoxo-

Cordelia

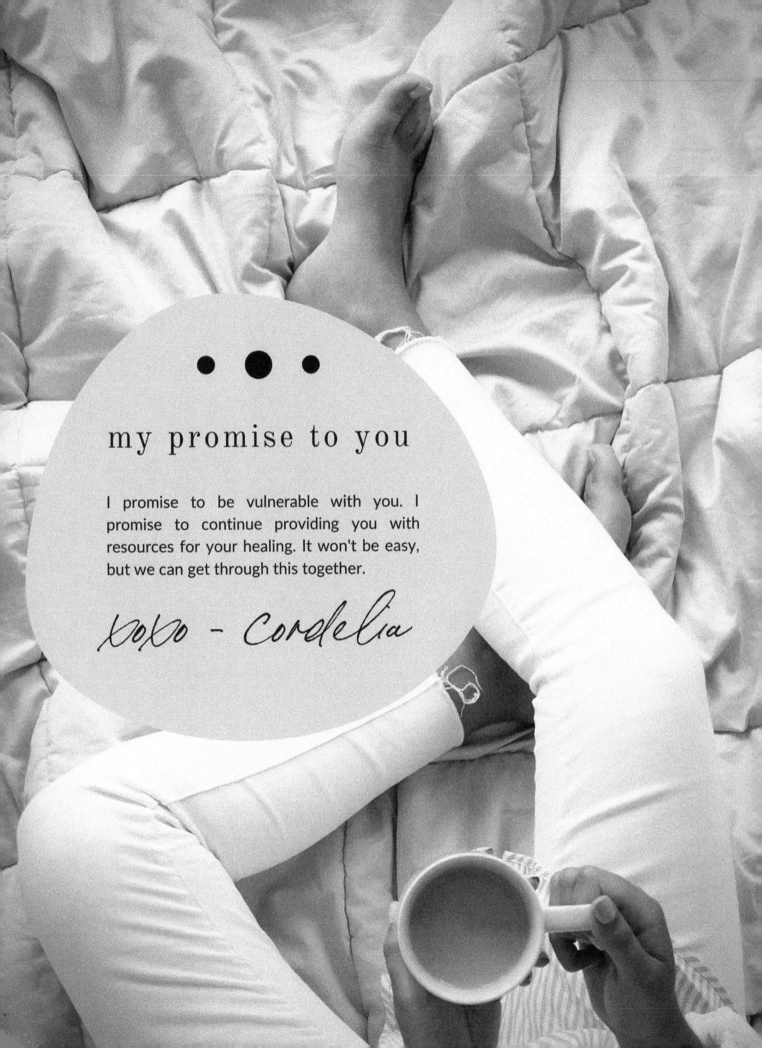

my promise to you

I promise to be vulnerable with you. I promise to continue providing you with resources for your healing. It won't be easy, but we can get through this together.

xoxo - Cordelia

let's set yourself up for success

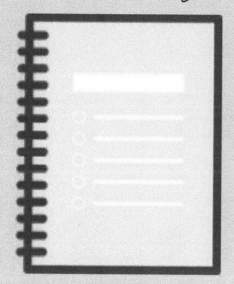

WHAT TO EXPECT: THE FIRST HALF

The first half of the workbook tackles four steps. Within each step, there are some baby steps.

- In step one, there is information about the science and research behind breakups. Additionally, there are questions and activities to help you process your breakup or divorce.
- In step two, there are straightforward actions for you to take to implement an action plan in healing from this experience.
- In step three, you will shift your focus to getting to know yourself, unpacking your underlying issues, and spending time thinking about your childhood.
- In step four, you will create your standards, such as boundaries and red flags.

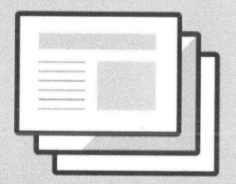

WHAT TO EXPECT: THE SECOND HALF

The second half of the workbook provides you with tools as you move forward with your life. You are given tips for breaking out of toxic relationship patterns, questions to ask yourself when you start dating again, and various resources that you may need in your healing journey.

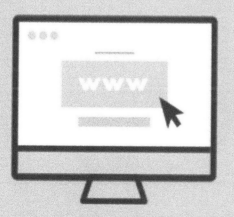

GET EXTRA HELP IF YOU NEED IT

Your healing journey does not need to end with this workbook. As mentioned, I have included tons of resources in this book. If you are still struggling, I encourage you to use those resources. As always, I also recommend finding a licensed counselor or medical professional to work through any issues that come up. If you already have a counselor, I encourage you to talk to your counselor about issues that come up for you as you do this workbook.

the healing roadmap

QUICK REFERENCE PAGE & TABLE OF CONTENTS

thinking ahead roadmap

PREFACE ● ● ●

He could smell me like sharks smell blood in the water. On our first date, I didn't realize I would spend the next 3.5 years of my life escaping him. Unsuspecting of the predator in front of me, I started to open up about myself as we got to know each other. As I peeled back the layers of me, his mask remained firmly in place. Months went by, and I couldn't hide who I was – giving, loving, hard-working, caring, kind. His mask stayed put.

I shared stories about my past. With each wound I unveiled to him, he noted the exact spot it healed so he could open it when he needed to revisit it. At the time, I didn't know I was handing over the blueprint to terrorize me.

As I told him about being put in the trunk of the car by my former partner, I never dreamed he would file that away in his brain to later use against me if I dared stand up to him. As I told him about past traumas and violations of my body, I never dreamed he would only use that information to manipulate me and wear down my spirit.

Sharks are typically viewed as apex predators and the top of the food chain. It is neither surprising nor shocking when a shark overcomes almost all of its prey. It is, however, impressive to learn about the prey that escapes the shark.

When Charles Darwin coined the phrase "survival of the fittest," I would like to think he was inspired by something similar to the prey overcoming the top predator. When the prey develops the ability to survive and not get eaten by the shark, this prey will be the one that evolves.

I didn't make this workbook for the sharks or the predators. I made this workbook for people like me - the prey that developed an ability to survive and not get eaten by the shark.

I hope this workbook helps you in your healing journey. Thank you for opening your heart and mind, and thank you for trusting me in your healing process.

xoxo- Cordelia

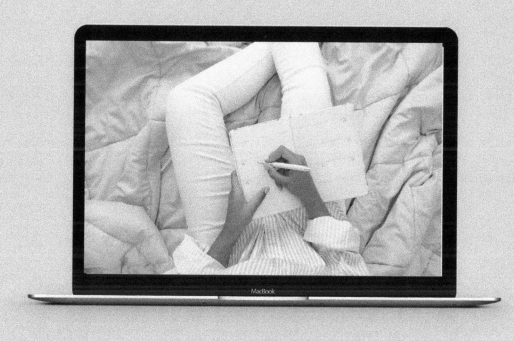

LET'S PROCESS
THE BREAKUP

● ● ●

STEP 1

step 1 roadmap
LET'S PROCESS THE BREAKUP

baby step 1
PAGE 7
The science behind a breakup with questions and reflection

baby step 2
PAGE 12
Questions to unpack your breakup

baby step 3
PAGE 18
Let's look at the receipts

baby step 4
PAGE 20
Self-reflection

"WE CAN DO HARD THINGS"

-GLENNON DOYLE, UNTAMED

baby step 1

• • •

THE SCIENCE BEHIND A BREAKUP WITH QUESTIONS FOR REFLECTION

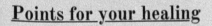

Key research

- *Breakups tend to happen for 8 reasons.*

- *We tend to drag out relationships that we otherwise would have ended when we are intertwined and have various commitments to the other person.*

Points for your healing

- *Consider the reasons your relationship ended.*

- *What, if any, commitments kept you in the relationship longer than you wanted?*

MOST BREAKUPS HAPPEN FOR THE FOLLOWING REASONS

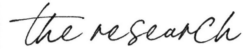

Research suggests most breakups happen due to the following reasons:

- ■ desire for more personal autonomy and independence
- ■ incompatibility (i.e. personality differences or not many common interests)
- ■ not feeling supported
- ■ lack of loyalty
- ■ not spending much time together
- ■ imbalance in fairness in the relationship
- ■ no romance in the relationship
- ■ lack of openness

Citation: Baxter, L. A. (1986). Gender Differences in the Hetero-Sexual Relationship Rules Embedded in Break-Up Accounts. Journal of Social and Personal Relationships, 3(3), 289–30
https://doi.org/10.1177/0265407586033003

Here are some factors that can drag out a relationship that you would have otherwise ended:

- ■ sharing a pet together
- ■ having a house together (or sharing a lease)
- ■ having future vacation plans together
- ■ sharing memberships or contracts (i.e. cell phone or gym)
- ■ being afraid to disappoint family or friends
- ■ sharing a joint bank account together
- ■ paying on each other's credit cards

Citation: Rhoades, G. K., Stanley, S. M., & Markman, H. J. (2010). Should I stay or should I go? Pred dating relationship stability from four aspects of commitment. Journal of family psychology : JFP : jour the Division of Family Psychology of the American Psychological Association (Division 43), 24(5), 543
https://doi.org/10.1037/a0021008

- *Breakups tend to follow the path mapped out on this page.*

- *Writing about your breakup or divorce has been shown to aid in healing.*

- *You should focus on trying to look at the experience in a new, positive lens.*

Points for your healing

- *What path did your breakup or divorce take?*

- *How long was the whole process? Try to find comfort in knowing that this was not a rash decision.*

- *Make it a goal to complete this workbook. Writing has been shown to help healing.*

MOST BREAKUPS FOLLOW A PATH
the research

Most breakups take the following path:

- loses interest in partner
- starts to notice other people
- starts to withdraw from the relationship
- tries to work it out
- starts spending less time with partner
- loses interest again
- tries to work it out again
- starts noticing other people again
- acts distant
- starts dating other people
- tries to work it out again with partner
- considers a breakup
- seriously distances themselves and starts testing waters of moving on
- breaks up

Citation: Battaglia DM, Richard FD, Datteri DL, Lord CG. Breaking Up is (Relatively) Easy to Do: A Script for the Dissolution of Close Relationships. Journal of Social and Personal Relationships. 1998;15(6):829-845. doi:10.1177/0265407598156007

THE PATH TO HEALING
the research

The following techniques have been shown to help in healing from a breakup or divorce:

- look at the breakup or divorce in a new, positive lens
- write about the positive facets of the breakup or divorce
- change your perspective
- shift focus to interpreting the experience in a more positive way

Citation: Lewandowski, G. W. (2009). Promoting positive emotions following relationship dissolution through writing. The Journal of Positive Psychology, 4(1), 21–31. https://doi.org/10.1080/17439760802068480

Key research

- *When we are rejected, the same area of our brain is triggered as when we experience physical pain.*

- *Human brains release natural painkillers in response to both physical pain and rejection.*

- *Love is an addiction. Our brain craves our ex, similar to how someone with an addiction craves drugs.*

Points for your healing

- *Your pain is valid.*

- *It is normal you are hurting.*

- *It is normal you feel addicted.*

- *You can boost your natural opioids.*

the research

Research has demonstrated that identical brain regions are activated in response to physical pain and in response to a breakup. In one study, researchers used functional magnetic resonance imaging ("functional MRI") in forty individuals who identified as feeling rejected after going through a breakup to test the hypothesis that breakup rejection can feel similar to physical pain. In the study, the participants viewed two sets of photographs (Kross et al., 2011). One collection of pictures were of their ex-partner, and the other was of a friend. While looking at the photographs of their ex-partner, they were instructed to think about how they felt during the breakup. While looking at their friend's pictures, they were told to think about a recent positive experience they shared with said friend.

To compare a breakup to physical pain, researchers used functional MRI in the same forty individuals to investigate how the brain reacts to a nonpainful situation and a painful situation. To create a painful condition, the researchers created a simulation where the participants felt like they spilled hot coffee on themselves. For the nonpainful situation, participants felt a nonpainful, warm, and thermal stimulation.

Bad breakups and the hot coffee sensation triggered the same regions of the brain. The researchers compared the areas of the brain that were being activated to over 500 studies. The majority of the 500 studies found identical regions were activated in response to physical pain. Thus, physical pain and breakups are registered in similar ways in our brains.

What has other research shown?

- The brain region called the anterior cingulate cortex (ACC) is activated when people feel physical pain and rejection (Eisenberger et al., 2003).

- The opioid response system, which releases natural painkillers, is activated in both physical pain and rejection (Hsu et al., 2013).

- Addiction studies show increased neurotransmitter dopamine in the nucleus accumbens are produced when someone craves drugs and when they think about an ex (Scofield et al., 2016).

Citations:
1. Kross, E., Berman, M. G., Mischel, W., Smith, E. E., & Wager, T. D. (2011). Social rejection shares somatosensory representations with physical pain. Proceedings of the National Academy of Sciences, 201102693. https://doi.org/10.1073/pnas.1102693108
2. Eisenberger, N. I., Lieberman, M. D., & Williams, K. D. (2003). Does Rejection Hurt? An fMRI Study of Social Exclusion. Science, 302(5643), 290. https://doi.org/10.1126/science.1089134
3. Hsu, D. T., Sanford, B. J., Meyers, K. K., Love, T. M., Hazlett, K. E., Wang, H., Ni, L., Walker, S. J., Mickey, B. J., Korycinski, S. T., Koeppe, R. A., Crocker, J. K., Langenecker, S. A., & Zubieta, J. K. (2013). Response of the μ-opioid system to social rejection and acceptance. Molecular psychiatry, 18(11), 1211–1217. https://doi.org/10.1038/mp.2013.96
4. Scofield, M. D., Heinsbroek, J. A., Gipson, C. D., Kupchik, Y. M., Spencer, S., Smith, A. C., Roberts-Wolfe, D., & Kalivas, P. W. (2016). The Nucleus Accumbens: Mechanisms of Addiction across Drug Classes Reflect the Importance of Glutamate Homeostasis. Pharmacological reviews, 68(3), 816–871. https://doi.org/10.1124/pr.116.012484

LET'S TALK ABOUT HOW YOU FEEL.

reflection.

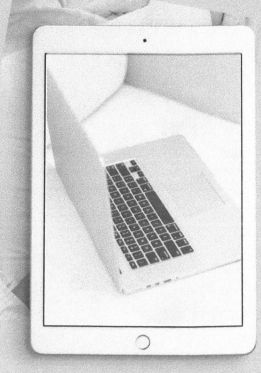

- ◼ Reflect on the research in this section.

- ◼ How do you feel about the research?

- ◼ How does your breakup compare?

- ◼ Reflect on all the questions presented throughout this section. You can write out your answers to those here as well.

TIME FOR REFLECTION

You can use the space below to write out your reflections. You may also use your computer or a sheet of paper. Follow the instructions at the top of the page for guidance on what to explore.

_____

_____

_____

_____

_____

_____

_____

_____

_____

_____

"EVEN IF THE MOST IMPORTANT PERSON IN YOUR WORLD REJECTS YOU, YOU ARE STILL REAL, AND YOU ARE STILL OKAY. IF YOU HAVE DONE SOMETHING INAPPROPRIATE OR YOU NEED TO SOLVE A PROBLEM OR CHANGE A BEHAVIOR, THEN TAKE APPROPRIATE STEPS TO TAKE CARE OF YOURSELF. BUT DON'T REJECT YOURSELF, AND DON'T GIVE SO MUCH POWER TO OTHER PEOPLE'S REJECTION OF YOU. IT ISN'T NECESSARY"

-MELODY BEATTIE, CODEPENDENT NO MORE

baby step 2

● ● ●

QUESTIONS TO UNPACK YOUR BREAKUP

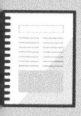

let's talk about your ex

The goal here is to dig into the relationship and your ex and look at the situation objectively.

INSTRUCTIONS

1 IN THIS SECTION, I WANT YOU TO SPEND TIME THINKING ABOUT THE QUESTIONS.

2 IF YOU NEED MORE SPACE, FEEL FREE TO ANSWER THE QUESTIONS ON YOUR COMPUTER, ON A PIECE OF PAPER, OR EVEN ON THE "NOTES" APP ON YOUR PHONE.

3 DON'T FEEL LIKE WRITING? ANSWER THE QUESTIONS OUT LOUD. YOU COULD EVEN RECORD YOUR ANSWERS SO YOU CAN LISTEN TO THEM AT A LATER DATE.

4 TRY TO ANSWER ALL QUESTIONS HONESTLY. NO ONE IS LOOKING OVER YOUR SHOULDER & CHECKING YOUR WORK.

How has your life improved since you & your ex broke up?

Tell me at least two things you learned from your relationship with your ex.

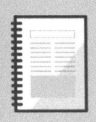

KEEP GOING, FRIEND.

What are the qualities you disliked about your ex?

What are some positives about being single?

What did you and your ex do when you spent time together?

What were the major issues in your relationship with your ex?

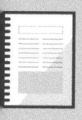

KEEP GOING, FRIEND.

Besides appearance, what are the qualities you liked about your ex?

How was the sex with your ex? How often did you orgasm? When you were intimate, do you feel like your ex cared about your enjoyment?

How did your ex treat you?

What are some parts of you that came out during the relationship that you would like to improve? What are some things you could have done better?

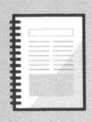

let's talk about your ex

How did your ex treat your friends and family?

Did you feel like your needs were met by your ex?

Did you become a better person at all in the course of the relationship? How so? Can you continue doing those things on your own?

Describe any current thoughts you have that hold you back from moving on from the relationship.

KEEP GOING, FRIEND.

How often did you cry in your relationship?

Who made the choice to end the relationship?

How can you grow from the relationship?

Describe the ways your ex felt familiar. (i.e., how was your ex similar to your previous dating partners, caregivers, etc.?)

"LET REALITY
BE REALITY."

- LAO TZU

baby step 3

● ● ●

LET'S LOOK AT THE RECEIPTS

LET'S LOOK AT THE RECEIPTS

what did your ex say?

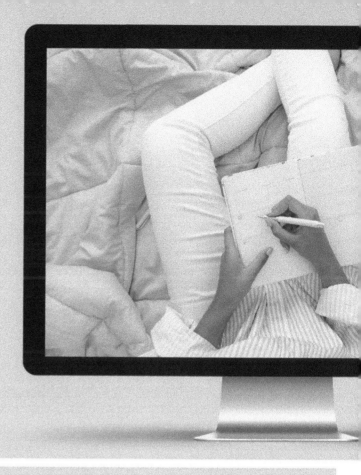

- When a relationship ends, we often romanticize it. That makes it hard to move on.

- I want you to look at your texts, emails, Facebook messages, or whatever communication you have between you two.

- What did your ex actually say to you? Was your ex nice? How did they treat you? What are the words that were said to you? How did the words make you feel?

WRITE IT OUT, FRIEND.

You can use the space below to write out your thoughts. You may also use your computer or a sheet of paper. Follow the instructions at the top of the page for guidance on what to explore.

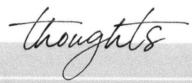

thoughts

"SUFFERING IS
PART OF LIFE.
MAY I BE KIND TO
MYSELF IN THIS
MOMENT.
MAY I GIVE MYSELF
THE COMPASSION
I NEED."

-KRISTIN NEFF, SELF-
COMPASSION: STOP BEATING
YOURSELF UP AND LEAVE
INSECURITY BEHIND

baby step 4

● ● ●

SELF-REFLECTION

LET'S LOOK INWARD

self-reflection

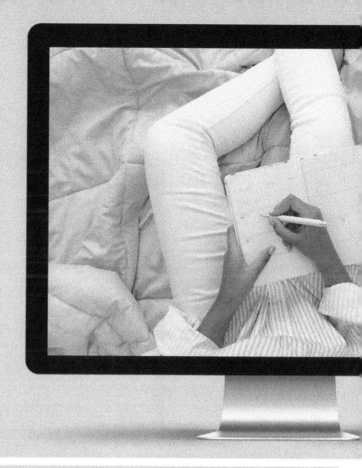

- ■ What aspects of the relationship are you still grieving?

- ■ What red flags did you ignore in the relationship? In what ways did you ignore the red flags, minimize them, or deny them?

- ■ Looking back, what boundaries should you have set in the relationship?

WRITE IT OUT, FRIEND.

You can use the space below to write out your thoughts. You may also use your computer or a sheet of paper. Follow the instructions at the top of the page for guidance on what to explore.

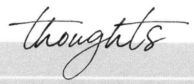

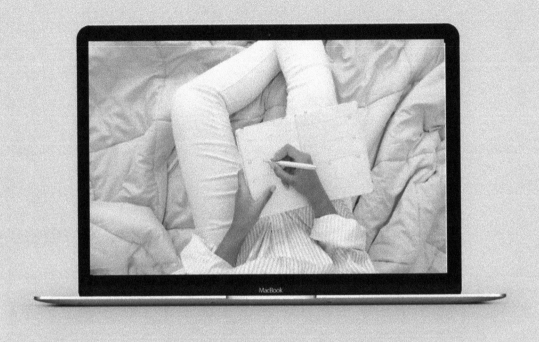

LET'S TAKE
SOME ACTIONS

● ● ●

STEP 2

step 2 roadMap
LET'S TAKE SOME ACTIONS

baby step 1
PAGE 24
Feel all your feelings

baby step 2
PAGE 27
Cut off contact with your ex
or utilize the gray rock method
and parallel parenting

baby step 3
PAGE 30
Accept that the relationship
is over

baby step 4
PAGE 32
Change how you talk
to yourself

baby step 5
PAGE 34
Change your thoughts

"IT'S OKAY TO FEEL ALL OF
THE STUFF YOU'RE FEELING.
YOU'RE JUST BECOMING
HUMAN AGAIN. YOU'RE NOT
DOING LIFE WRONG; YOU'RE
DOING IT RIGHT. IF THERE'S
ANY SECRET YOU'RE MISSING,
IT'S THAT DOING IT RIGHT IS
JUST REALLY HARD. FEELING
ALL YOUR FEELINGS IS HARD,
BUT THAT'S WHAT THEY'RE
FOR. FEELINGS ARE FOR
FEELING. ALL OF THEM. EVEN
THE HARD ONES. THE SECRET
IS THAT YOU'RE DOING IT
RIGHT, AND THAT DOING IT
RIGHT HURTS SOMETIMES."

-GLENNON DOYLE, UNTAMED

baby step 1

● ● ●

FEEL YOUR FEELINGS

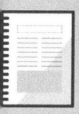

name your feelings

We have to be able to name our feelings in order to process what we are feeling.

1

NAME YOUR FEELINGS

PRACTICE naming your feelings and emotions. If you find yourself frequently saying "I"m fine" and numbing your emotions, try to make a conscious effort to begin naming your feelings.

2

DIG DEEPER THAN PRIMARY EMOTIONS + EXPAND YOUR EMOTIONAL VOCABULARY

How often do you simply say "sad" or "happy" when stating how you feel? Do you tend to not dig much deeper? I challenge you to start using more precise language and expand your emotional vocabulary. I want you to start using more words to describe how you are feeling. If you limit your emotions to just a few words, you can see how you ultimately limit your understanding of your emotions and numb out the wide range of emotions you are feeling.

3

PAY ATTENTION TO HOW YOUR BODY PHYSICALLY FEELS

For example, in my personal experience, I never used to put much thought into headaches, stomachaches, etc. These can really correlate to how you are doing emotionally.

4

USE A VOCABULARY OF EMOTIONS PDF, FEELINGS WHEEL, OR EMOTION-SENSATION FEELING WHEEL

I've listed resources below.

RECOMMENDED RESOURCES

Tom Drummond's Vocabulary of Emotions PDF
Free PDF. He compiled synonyms and other words for common primary emotions we express.

Gottman's Feeling Wheel
Useful tool in naming & recognizing emotions.

Lindsay Braman's Emotion-Sensation Feeling Wheel
This adds an additional layer to the traditional feelings wheel, and it help you think about what physical sensations you are feeing.

tip

Screenshot these on your phone or print them out to keep handy to practice using different words when determining how you feel.

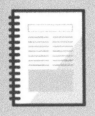

let's reflect on your feelings

LET'S BE REAL, FRIEND.

Have you tried to numb your feelings at all? If so, describe how. Some examples are drinking alcohol, binge eating, and staying busy.

How have you judged your emotions? ("I shouldn't be feeling this way," "I am being weak," etc.)

What words do you tend to use to describe your feelings or emotions?

What is something you can say to yourself when you feel yourself trying to suppress your feelings?

tips

■ Pay attention to how y◆ talk to yourself.

■ Remind yourself: "It's okay to feel like this."

"WHEN YOU NOTICE
SOMEONE DOES
SOMETHING TOXIC
THE FIRST TIME,
DON'T WAIT FOR THE
SECOND TIME BEFORE
YOU ADDRESS IT OR
CUT THEM OFF."

— SHAHIDA ARABI

baby step 2

• • •

CUT OFF CONTACT WITH YOUR EX

OR

UTILIZE THE GRAY ROCK METHOD
& PARALLEL PARENTING

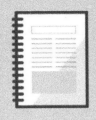

1

GO NO CONTACT

If possible, change your number. You should delete your ex off all social media, block their number, and don't respond to any form of communication from them.

2

THERE IS NOTHING TO TALK ABOUT

There are no further discussions you need to have with your ex. By reaching out to your ex after a breakup, you are chipping away at your self-esteem. By maintaining contact, you are sending the following messages to yourself and to your ex: (1) "I don't know how to live without this person," (2) "Even after this person broke my heart, I still want them in my life," (3) "I'm available, even though this person is clearly not emotionally available for a relationship."

3

IF YOU ABSOLUTELY CANNOT CUT OFF CONTACT (I.E., YOU SHARE CUSTODY OF A CHILD), YOU MUST USE THE GRAY ROCK METHOD AND PARALLEL PARENTING

Check out the information below for an overview of what those are.
Let's make one thing very clear, though: This should only be done if you actually have ZERO options of going no contact.

GRAY ROCK METHOD

- **Gray Rock is how it sounds**
  You become a gray rock. In other words, you become a dull, monotonous, emotionless person when it comes to your ex.

- **Offer no explanations or defenses**
  Do not explain yourself or defend yourself to your ex.

- **Keep answers short, preferably one word**
  "Yes," "no," or "I don't know"

- **Avoid eye contact**
  When you make eye contact with someone, you can form an emotional connection, so try to look elsewhere.

- **Avoid communicating verbally or in person**
  Try to avoid phone calls or in-person talks. All communication should be done over email, text, or another form of writing.

- **Don't give your ex details about your life**
  Don't tell them about your dating life or anything else.

- **Don't try to hold your ex accountable**
  Don't try to talk to them about how they have hurt you or anything else emotional.

PARALLEL PARENTING

- **Parents detach + choose how to parent**
  Parents detach from one another. Each parent chooses how to raise the child while said parent is responsible for taking care of them.

- **Considerably different from co-parenting**
  Co-parenting is where two healthy adults can come together to raise their child, despite differences between them.

- **Everything is separate**
  Parents attend nothing together.

- **Parallel parenting is recommended in certain situations**
  It is recommended where one of the parents has been abusive, borderline personality disorder, or narcissistic personality disor[der]

- **It does not have to be permanent**
  You can simply use this as a tool until you have healed and are [with] the other parent.

  Check out www.ourfamilywizard.com. You can put schedules on there, as well as child's medical info, educational info, and babysitter info. You can also communicate there.

Citations
1. Harrigan, E. (2015, December 06). Parallel Parenting. Retrieved September 18, 2020, from https://outofthefog.website/separating-divorcing/2015/12/6/parallel-parenting
2. Raypole, C. (2019, December 13). Grey Rock Method: 6 Tips and Techniques. Retrieved September 18, 2020, from https://www.healthline.com/health/grey-rock

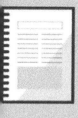

LET'S BE REAL, FRIEND.

What is keeping you from implementing the no-contact rule or gray rock method?

How is not implementing the no-contact rule or gray rock method keeping you from healing?

How can you give yourself permission to implement the no-contact rule or gray rock method?

What is something you can say to yourself when you feel overwhelmed, anxious, guilty, or sad about going no contact or utilizing gray rock method?

tips

- You are strong enough to do this.

- It will be hard, and you may be sad at first. That's okay. Allow yourself to be sad.

"HAPPINESS
CAN EXIST
ONLY IN
ACCEPTANCE."

-GEORGE ORWELL

baby step 3

• • •

ACCEPT THAT THE RELATIONSHIP IS OVER

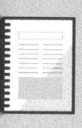

First, you should read over the tips about accepting that it's over. Next, you should use the space below to give yourself permission to release the relationship and accept that it's over. Write whatever comes to your heart.

face reality

it's over

1 — FACE REALITY

It's normal to be in denial initially. However, acceptance is an essential part of healing, and you cannot fight it for long. You have to face reality and face yourself. Acknowledge it is over.

2 — SAY IT WITH ME: "WHAT WE HAD IS FINISHED."

..and say it over and over again. It's over and finished. The only step from here is to continue down the road in front of you and to stop looking backward.

3 — GET RID OF ALL REMINDERS OF YOUR EX

Take down all pictures of your ex (even ones on your phone), gifts they gave you, their hoodie you still sleep in, or anything that reminds you of them. I started a fire and burnt all our pictures, but hey, whatever works for you.

release the relationship

"DON'T WAIT ON
ANYONE TO TELL
YOU WHAT YOU ARE
WORTH. YOU HAVE TO
BE THE FIRST PERSON
WHO KNOWS WHAT
YOU ARE WORTH AND
CAN SAY WHAT YOU
ARE WORTH."

-CLEO WADE, HEART TALK:
POETIC WISDOM FOR
A BETTER LIFE

baby step 4

● ● ●

CHANGE HOW YOU TALK TO YOURSELF

• • •

Key points

- *How we talk to ourselves matters.*

- *In therapy for depression, one of the critical things therapists work on is shifting negative self-talk to positive self-talk.*

- *You can practice incorporating positive self-talk into your life.*

• • •

Tips for talking to yourself more positively

- *Pay attention to how you are talking to yourself.*

- *Use the tips you will learn in baby step #5 to work on your thoughts.*

- *Try out some positive affirmations.*

CHANGE HOW YOU TALK TO YOURSELF

the basics

Self-talk is "verbalizations or statements addressed to the self" (Hardy, 2006). In more simple terms, it is "the way your inner voice makes sense of the world around you and the way you communicate with your inner self" (Scott, 2020). Self-talk can be negative or positive.

As Gregory L. Jantz, Ph.D. writes:

"Too often, the pattern of self-talk we've developed is negative. We remember the negative things we were told as children by our parents, siblings, or teachers. We remember the negative reactions from other children that diminished how we felt about ourselves. Throughout the years, these messages have played over and over in our minds, fueling our feelings of anger, fear, guilt, and hopelessness. One of the most critical avenues we use in therapy with those suffering from depression is to identify the source of these messages and then work with the person to intentionally "overwrite" them. If a person learned as a child, he was worthless, we show him how truly special he is. If, while growing up, a person learned to expect crises and destructive events, we show her a better way to anticipate the future" (Jantz, 2016).

Unsurprisingly, the research overwhelmingly suggests the way we talk to ourselves greatly impacts our lives.

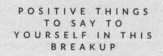

POSITIVE THINGS TO SAY TO YOURSELF IN THIS BREAKUP

- ■ I will love again.
- ■ It's over and I can handle that.
- ■ It's okay to be sad that it's over.
- ■ I can learn from this experience.
- ■ This is hard to go through.
- ■ I've been through breakups before, and I can survive this.

- ■ I can take this as slow as I need.
- ■ It feels hard to admit it's over.
- ■ It will get easier to admit it's over.
- ■ I am choosing a healthy direction.
- ■ It's okay if I need to cry.
- ■ I have coping skills I can use to get through this, and I can always call my counselor to schedule an appointment.

Citations:
1. Hardy, J. (2006). Speaking clearly: A critical review of the self-talk literature. Psychology of Sport and Exercise, 7, 81-97.
2. Jantz, G. L., Ph.D. (2016, May 16). The Power of Positive Self-Talk. Retrieved September 20, 2020, from https://www.psychologytoday.com/us/blog/hope-relationships/201605/the-power-positive-self-talk
3. Scott, E., MS. (2020, July 20). Positive Self Talk for a Better Life. Retrieved September 20, 2020, from https://www.verywellmind.com/how-to-use-positive-self-talk-for-stress-relief-3144816

"WHETHER YOU
THINK YOU CAN,
OR YOU THINK
YOU CAN'T--
YOU'RE RIGHT."

-HENRY FORD

baby step 5

● ● ●

CHANGE YOUR THOUGHTS

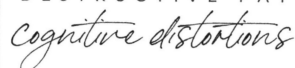

Cognitive distortions

Cognitive distortions are biased, negative, and automatic ways of thinking about ourselves, other people, and the world around us. They are typically related to our beliefs about ourselves. These thinking patterns can cause us to spiral out of control, and it's super important to spend time transforming these maladaptive ways of thinking.

Here are examples of cognitive distortions as they would look in a breakup:

- **All-or-nothing thinking:** There is no middle ground. You are either perfect or a failure (i.e. ,"If I get divorced, I am worthless and a failure").

- **Overgeneralization:** You use words like always, never, everybody, and no one (i.e. , "No one will ever want to date me again").

- **Dwelling on the negative**: You focus on one negative and exclude all positives (i.e., "He rejected me, so I will never enjoy my life again").

- **Rejecting the positive:** You refuse to embrace any positive (i.e., you get asked out by someone and say, "Oh, they just asked me out because they feel sorry for me").

- **Assuming the worst**: You assume the worst about what someone is thinking or what their intentions are (i.e., "I know he hates me").

- **Fortune telling**: You act like you are able to predict the future, despite that being impossible (i.e., "I will never find love again").

- **Catastrophizing**: You expect the worst to happen, and it's typically something that has almost no chance of happening (i.e., "I will die if we break up").

- **Feelings = facts**: You feel a feeling and decide it is a fact (i.e., "I feel ugly, so I am ugly").

- **The "Shoulds"**: You demand yourself to meet an expectation or a timeline, and you shame yourself for not meeting it (i.e. "I should be over this").

- **Labeling**: When you feel a certain way or when something negative happens, you define yourself based on this one emotion (i.e., "I am worthless").

- **Personalization**: You take everything personally, and you take events as definitions of your worth (i.e., "If only I didn't annoy him, he wouldn't call me names").

- **Fallacy of fairness**: You expect life to be fair, and you expect the world to treat you fairly (i.e., "It is not fair we are breaking up").

- **Fallacy of change**: You believe if certain people or things would change, you would finally be happy (i.e., "If he would just change, we'd be happy").

- **Blaming**: Nothing is ever your fault, and you are never wrong. You are the helpless victim (i.e., "I did absolutely nothing wrong").

- **Heaven's reward fallacy**: You believe you should be rewarded based on what you've done (i.e., "I put six years into this relationship, and I deserve a happy ending with him").

Citations:
1. Rnic, K., Dozois, D. J., & Martin, R. A. (2016). Cognitive Distortions, Humor Styles, and Depression. Europe's journal of psychology, 12(3), 348–362. https://doi.org/10.5964/ejop.v12i3.1118
2. Ackerman, C. (2020, September 01). Cognitive Distortions: When Your Brain Lies to You (+ PDF Worksheets). Retrieved September 20, 2020, from https://positivepsychology.com/cognitive-distortions/

starting point for when ● ● ●
you experience these
types of thoughts..

questions to ask

■ What am I feeling right now physically?

■ What am I feeling right now mentally?

■ Did anything in particular trigger this thought?

■ Does a particular person trigger this thought?

■ What did I do last time I felt like this?
Did it help?

■ Have I ever thought like this before?

■ Am I acting like I could have controlled
the situation or the outcome?

■ What was I aware of at the time?

■ Am I holding myself to an impossible
standard?

■ Am I expecting more of myself than
I would of a loved one?

■ Does thinking like this serve me in any way?

■ What would it feel like if I choose to think
about this in a more positive way?

■ How would I soothe a friend who was
having thoughts like this?

■ What is one thing I can do to step out of
this cycle?

■ What can I do different when I feel
this in the future?

■ Am I having trouble processing
this on my own?

■ Should I call a loved one to talk things out?

■ Should I make an appointment with a
counselor, psychiatrist, or professional?

Over the next few pages,
there are more specific examples
of questions for common thoughts
you may have in a breakup.

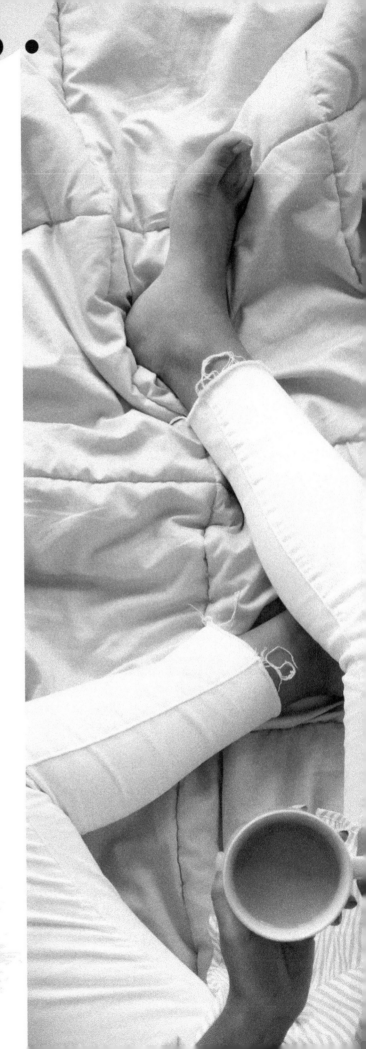

"It's all my fault."

1

QUESTION

Am I trying to make my feeling into a fact?

2

QUESTION

Am I really 100% at fault?

3

QUESTION

Is it possible I'm less than 100% at fault?

4

QUESTION

If I assume everything is my fault, what is the worst possible outcome?

5

QUESTION

Do I think it's my fault just because someone told me it was?

6

QUESTION

Why do I think everything is my fault?

7

QUESTION

What evidence is there that this is not 100% my fault?

8

QUESTION

Have I already accepted responsibility for what I did wrong?

9

QUESTION

What positive impact is dwelling on this having on my life?

"I'm worthless."

WHEN YOU HAVE THIS THOUGHT...

In addition to the list I previously provided, these specific questions may be helpful for you.

QUESTION 1

Why do I think I'm worthless?

QUESTION 2

What evidence is there that I'm not worthless?

QUESTION 3

Where is this thought coming from?

QUESTION 4

What is the first memory I have of thinking I'm worthless?

QUESTION 5

How long have I called myself worthless?

QUESTION 6

Am I going through a tough time and need some help coping?

QUESTION 7

Am I only thinking this because someone told me I'm worthless?

QUESTION 8

If someone called me worthless, is it possible they were projecting onto me?

QUESTION 9

If I heard my friend call themself worthless, would it make me sad?

"I will never fall in love again."

In addition to the list I previously provided, these specific questions may be helpful for you.

QUESTION 1

Am I using words like always, never, everybody, and nobody?

QUESTION 2

Am I exaggerating?

QUESTION 3

What would it feel like to use more specific language (like "I might fall in love again or I might not")?

QUESTION 4

Do I have the power to see into the future?

QUESTION 5

How do I know I will never fall in love again?

QUESTION 6

Isn't it possible I could fall in love again?

QUESTION 7

Isn't it possible I could meet someone amazing one day?

QUESTION 8

How is this thought serving me in a positive way?

QUESTION 9

What would I say to a friend who said they would never fall in love again?

"If I'd just had sex more, my ex wouldn't have cheated."

WHEN YOU HAVE THIS THOUGHT...

In addition to the list I previously provided, these specific questions may be helpful for you.

1

QUESTION

Am I acting like I had the power to control another person?

2

QUESTION

If I did just have sex more, how do I know they wouldn't have cheated?

3

QUESTION

Isn't it possible they cheated for other reasons?

4

QUESTION

Why would I want to be in a relationship where I can't be myself?

5

QUESTION

Why would I want to be in a relationship where I have to do things to keep my partner from cheating?

6

QUESTION

What can I do right now to take a step toward living in the present?

7

QUESTION

Am I avoiding grieving the relationship?

8

QUESTION

If I had a healthy relationship, would my partner cheat on me for this reason?

9

QUESTION

How can I accept the possibility that I may never know why my ex cheated on me?

"If my relationship ends, I am a failure."

WHEN YOU HAVE THIS THOUGHT...

In addition to the list I previously provided, these specific questions may be helpful for you.

QUESTION 1

Aren't there other parts of me besides my relationship?

QUESTION 2

If my relationship ends, does that mean all the other parts of me also end?

QUESTION 3

Why am I deeming myself a failure when I have other things going for me?

QUESTION 4

Isn't it fair to say I've tried hard in the relationship?

QUESTION 5

Is it possible this relationship just wasn't right for me?

QUESTION 6

Why am I calling myself a name due to a relationship not working out?

QUESTION 7

If I wasted my life in an unhappy relationship, would that be more or less of a "fail"?

QUESTION 8

Why am I acting like my worth is proportional to this relationship?

QUESTION 9

Is there another way I can think about this?

"If we aren't together, I can't survive."

WHEN YOU HAVE THIS THOUGHT...

In addition to the list I previously provided, these specific questions may be helpful for you.

1
QUESTION

What are the chances I will actually die from this relationship ending?

2
QUESTION

If we can't be together, what can I do?

3
QUESTION

In twenty years, will I care about this?

4
QUESTION

Have I survived previous breakups before this one?

5
QUESTION

Is it possible I am exaggerating?

6
QUESTION

Is this triggering any feelings of abandonment for me?

7
QUESTION

What other things in my life do I have going for me outside of this person?

8
QUESTION

What are some new things I could try in my spare time?

9
QUESTION

Are there any friends or family I could call to talk to about things?

"Nobody wants to be with me."

WHEN YOU HAVE THIS THOUGHT...

In addition to the list I previously provided, these specific questions may be helpful for you.

1

QUESTION

Am I using the word nobody?

2

QUESTION

Am I exaggerating?

3

QUESTION

What would it feel like to use more specific language (like "some people want to be with me and some don't")?

4

QUESTION

Since I've dated people before, wouldn't that mean there are people that have wanted to be with me?

5

QUESTION

If I've dated before, why do I think no one will continue wanting to date me?

6

QUESTION

How do I know who will want to date me in the future?

7

QUESTION

Where is this thought coming from?

8

QUESTION

When is the first time I remember thinking something like this?

9

QUESTION

What can I do to show myself some compassion?

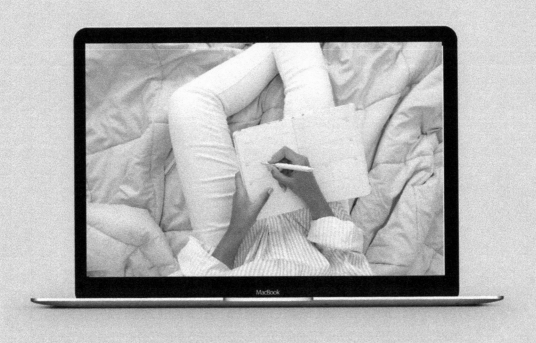

LET'S GET TO KNOW YOU

• • •

STEP 3

step 3 roadMap

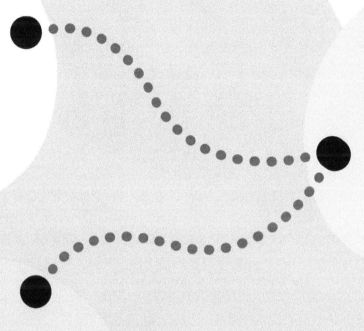

baby step 1

PAGE 46

Questions to help figure out
who you are

baby step 2

PAGE 55

Reflecting on your family of
origin

baby step 3

PAGE 58

Letter to your inner child

"IF YOU DON'T KNOW WHO YOU ARE, YOU ARE GOING TO THINK SOMEONE ELSE'S DESCRIPTION ACCURATELY DESCRIBES YOU."

- CORDELIA

baby step!

● ● ●

QUESTIONS TO FIGURE OUT WHO YOU ARE

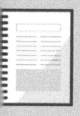

questions to help figure out
who you are

1 IN THIS SECTION, I WANT YOU TO SPEND TIME THINKING ABOUT THE QUESTIONS.

2 IF YOU NEED MORE SPACE, FEEL FREE TO ANSWER THE QUESTIONS ON YOUR COMPUTER, ON A PIECE OF PAPER, OR EVEN ON THE "NOTES" APP ON YOUR PHONE.

3 DON'T FEEL LIKE WRITING? ANSWER THE QUESTIONS OUT LOUD. YOU COULD EVEN RECORD YOUR ANSWERS SO YOU CAN LISTEN TO THEM AT A LATER DATE.

4 TRY TO ANSWER ALL QUESTIONS HONESTLY. NO ONE IS LOOKING OVER YOUR SHOULDER & CHECKING YOUR WORK.

What do you like to do in your free time?

Who do you like to spend your time with?

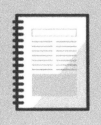

KEEP GOING, FRIEND.

Where do you work? How did you end up working there?

What is your educational background? What led you down that particular path?

What are you skilled or talented in?

What are your spiritual or religious beliefs? How did you come into those beliefs?

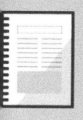

questions to help figure out

who you are

What are you passionate about? What sets your soul on fire?

How do you hope you are remembered by others?

What do you want to do most with your remaining time on this planet?

What part of you do you hide from others? Why?

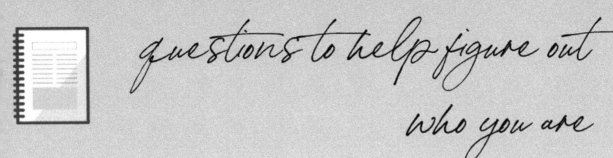

questions to help figure out who you are

What are your three best qualities?

What is your dream career?

What character traits do you admire in other people?

What are beliefs you have about yourself that are holding you back?

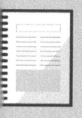

questions to help figure out who you are

How can you give yourself permission to stop worrying about what others think of you?

What does success look like to you?

How can you enjoy today more?

What can you start doing to begin accepting who you are?

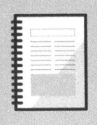

questions to help figure out

who you are

What makes you lose track of time?

Who are the one or two people you admire the most?

What are some compliments you have received?

What hard things have you faced in your life?

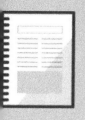

questions to help figure out
who you are

Name some things you are good at.

What is your favorite thing about your appearance?

What emotions do you fight with and try to get rid of?

What memories, thoughts, or fears do you find yourself dwelling on or obsessing over?

KEEP GOING, FRIEND.

What are you currently doing that makes your life worse?

How would you like to grow as a person?

What hobby would you do if you had all the time in the world?

How could you use your talents to help others in the world?

"FOR IN EVERY ADULT THERE DWELLS THE CHILD THAT WAS, AND IN EVERY CHILD THERE LIES THE ADULT THAT WILL BE."

-JOHN CONNOLLY, THE BOOK OF LOST THINGS

baby step 2

• • •

REFLECTING ON YOUR FAMILY OF ORIGIN

how did your caregivers
show up for you?

You can either: (1) use the questions below as journal prompts and write out responses on a separate sheet of paper, (2) think through the questions in your head, or (3) talk through the questions out loud to yourself.

QUESTION

How did your caregivers model apologies when you grew up?

QUESTION

What role did you play in your family growing up?

QUESTION

Were you designated as the problem child?

QUESTION

Were you deemed the golden child?

QUESTION

Were you forgotten about?

QUESTION

How often were you blamed by your caregiver?

QUESTION

Did you have any sense of autonomy as a child?

QUESTION

What parts of you do you feel like your caregiver resented?

QUESTION

Did you feel unworthy as a child?

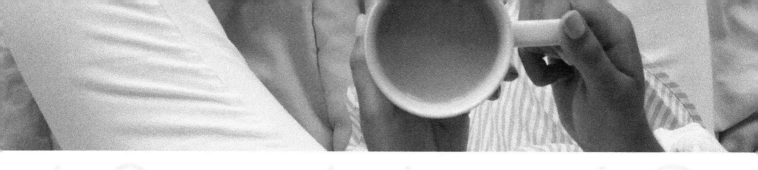

10

QUESTION

What did you need your caregivers to do as a child?

11

QUESTION

How did your caregivers give gifts as child? Were you ever made to feel unappreciative upon receipt?

12

QUESTION

Did your caregivers respect your boundaries as a child?

13

QUESTION

When you were little, did you ever try to run away from home? What made you want to leave?

14

QUESTION

What names did your caregivers call you as a child?

15

QUESTION

What sayings, expressions, or advice did you hear your caregivers say when you were growing up?

16

QUESTION

Did your caregivers put a lot of pressure on your grades?

17

QUESTION

Did your caregivers have friends? How did your caregivers model friendship?

18

QUESTION

Did your caregivers take you on play dates and create an environment where you would have friends?

"SHE HELD HERSELF UNTIL THE SOBS OF THE CHILD INSIDE SUBSIDED ENTIRELY. I LOVE YOU, SHE TOLD HERSELF. IT WILL ALL BE OKAY."

-H. RAVEN ROSE, SHADOW SELVES: DOUBLE HAPPINESS

baby step 3

• • •

LETTER TO YOUR INNER CHILD

WRITE A
LETTER TO
your inner child

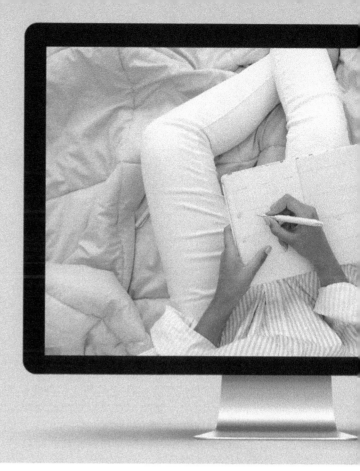

Imagine you are able to send a letter back in time to your inner child. Tell your inner child that you are *you* from the future. Tell your inner child how you know their pain, struggles, sadness, and issues. Tell your inner child all the things they lack from their childhood. Tell your inner child it's not their fault.

You may use the space below or another method if you prefer.

thoughts

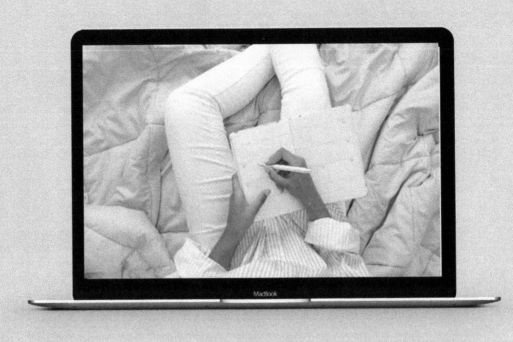

LET'S ESTABLISH OUR BASELINES

• • •

STEP 4

our baselines

THE ESSENTIALS

"COMPASSIONATE PEOPLE ASK FOR WHAT THEY NEED. THEY SAY NO WHEN THEY NEED TO, AND WHEN THEY SAY YES THEY MEAN IT. THEY'RE COMPASSIONATE BECAUSE THEIR BOUNDARIES KEEP THEM OUT OF RESENTMENT."

- BRENÉ BROWN, RISING STRONG

baseline #1

● ● ●

LET'S SET YOUR BOUNDARIES

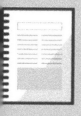

let's set your boundaries.

How do the people around you treat you? Be sure to think about various people such as your friends, family members, significant others, etc.

How do you respond when anyone treats you badly?

Do you feel worthy of having needs? Why or why not?

Describe a time you've tried to set a boundary and failed. What happened? Why did it fail?

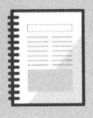

let's set your boundaries.

Who do you struggle setting boundaries with?

Why do you struggle settling boundaries with these people?

What is something you can do today to take a step toward enforcing your boundaries?

What are two things you can do this month to take steps toward enforcing your boundaries?

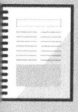

let's set your boundaries.

Do you feel anxiety about setting a boundary? Where is that feeling coming from?

What holds you back from setting a boundary?

Do you feel worthy enough to set a boundary? If not, what makes you think your needs are unimportant?

you set a boundary and the other person does not respect it, what are you prepared to do?

Your Boundaries

| # 1 | # 2 | # 3 | # 4 | # 5 | # 6 |

| # 7 | # 8 | # 9 | # 10 | # 11 | # 12 |

| # 13 | # 14 | # 15 | # 16 | # 17 | # 18 |

| # 19 | # 20 | # 21 | # 22 | # 23 | # 24 |

you can do this.

"RED FLAGS ARE
MOMENTS OF
HESITATION THAT
DETERMINE OUR
DESTINATION."

-MANDY HALE, THE SINGLE
WOMAN: LIFE, LOVE, AND A DASH
OF SASS

baseline #2

● ● ●

LET'S FIGURE OUT WHAT YOUR RED FLAGS ARE

Cordelia's Red Flags

These are just some of my red flags that I've noted from my experience. Read this over before going to the next page to work on your list.

#1

Potential partner ("PP") is rude to wait staff.

#2

PP drinks every time we hang out.

#3

PP smokes weed every day.

#4

PP never says sorry.

#5

PP says all their exes are crazy.

#6

PP starts talking about "our future" very early on.

#7

PP seemingly has no boundaries with their parents.

#8

PP stops planning stuff for us to do after first few months.

#9

PP wants me to change things about myself.

#10

PP always expects me to hang out at their place, and PP never makes an effort to come to mine.

#11

PP tries to shame me in any way.

#12

PP raises their voice at me during a conflict.

#13

PP doesn't carry condoms, doesn't discuss birth control, and doesn't discuss STD testing.

#14

PP tries to isolate me from friends or family.

#15

PP isn't there when I need them (i.e. need ride to hospital and doesn't help).

#16

PP talks about their ex a lot.

#17

PP doesn't buy or order my birthday present. Asks me to order what I want and they'll pay me.

#18

PP desperately wants their parents' approval

#19

PP uses the phrase "all women do" followed by a blanket generalization.

#20

PP tells me what a good person they are.

#21

PP storms off in middle of fight and disappears for nights or days.

#22

PP engages in silent treatment.

#23

PP gets mad at me over something I did accidently (i.e. broke a glass).

#24

PP has different personalities aroun different people (i.e huge parts of their life that others don know about).

you Can do this.

Your
Red Flags

1   # 2   # 3   # 4   # 5   # 6

7   # 8   # 9   # 10   # 11   # 12

13   # 14   # 15   # 16   # 17   # 18

19   # 20   # 21   # 22   # 23   # 24

you can do this.

"YOU GET WHAT YOU TOLERATE."

-HENRY CLOUD, BOUNDARIES IN MARRIAGES

baseline #3

• • •

LET'S SET YOUR "STRIKE ONE & YOU'RE OUTS"

Cordelia's Strike One & You're Outs

"Strike One & You're Outs" are your non-negotiables. If any of these happen, you walk away from this person. Think of it like this: If X happens, then I'm gone.

Here is my list to get you started.

 # 1
Potential Partner ("PP") calls me mes.

 # 2
If PP cheats on me.

 # 3
If I have no shared interests with PP.

 # 4
If I have no shared values with PP.

 # 5
If PP never acknowledges their faults.

 # 6
If I don't feel safe around PP.

 # 7
PP is consistent.

 # 8
If I don't feel comfortable being myself around PP.

 # 9
If PP does not respect my boundaries.

 # 10
If PP does not add value to my life.

 # 11
If PP's words and actions don't match.

 # 12
If PP does not plan dates and stuff for us to do.

 # 13
PP does not communicate well.

 # 14
If PP is pining over an ex.

 # 15
If PP never makes me laugh.

 # 16
If PP does not admit when they are wrong.

 # 17
If PP does not follow through on things they say they will do.

 # 18
If PP has no boundaries with their own parents.

 # 19
PP does not like ogs.

 # 20
If PP does not treat my dogs well.

 # 21
If PP expects me to clean, cook, and take care of them.

 # 22
If PP does not know how to control their anger.

 # 23
If PP tries to make me feel crazy.

 # 24
If PP engages in silent treatment or goes MIA.

you can do this.

Your
Strike One &
You're Outs

• • •

1   # 2   # 3   # 4   # 5   # 6

7   # 8   # 9   # 10   # 11   # 12

13   # 14   # 15   # 16   # 17   # 18

19   # 20   # 21   # 22   # 23   # 24

you can do this.

"YOUR PERSONAL
BOUNDARIES
PROTECT THE INNER
CORE OF YOUR
IDENTITY AND YOUR
RIGHT TO CHOICES."

- GERARD MANLEY HOPKINS

baseline #4

● ● ●

YOUR BARE MINIMUMS

Cordelia's
Bare Minimums

Bare minimums are the lowest bar that you will accept from a person.

I'm sharing my list for you to get some ideas in creating yours.

 # 1
Potential partner ("PP") must have a job.

 # 2
I must be attracted to PP.

 # 3
I must enjoy talking to PP.

 # 4
PP must be kind.

 # 5
PP must not have an active substance abuse problem (i.e. alcohol, drugs).

 # 6
PP must not have a mental illness they are neglecting (i.e. not seeing a counselor, etc).

 # 7
PP must have basic empathy and manners.

 # 8
PP must live within their means.

 # 9
PP must not smoke weed daily.

 # 10
PP must be a hard worker.

 # 11
PP must know how to control their anger.

 # 12
PP must make me feel safe and respected.

 # 13
PP must be honest.

 # 14
PP must plan dates.

 # 15
PP must communicate well.

 # 16
PP must not be pining over an ex.

 # 17
PP must make me laugh.

 # 18
PP must admit when they are wrong.

 # 19
PP must follow through on their word.

 # 20
PP must have boundaries with parents.

 # 21
PP must not expect me to clean, cook, and take care of them.

 # 22
PP must not call me names.

 # 23
PP must like dogs & be good to my dogs.

 # 24
PP must add value to my life.

you can do this.

Your
Bare Minimums

| # 1 | # 2 | # 3 | # 4 | # 5 | # 6 |

| # 7 | # 8 | # 9 | # 10 | # 11 | # 12 |

| # 13 | # 14 | # 15 | # 16 | # 17 | # 18 |

| # 19 | # 20 | # 21 | # 22 | # 23 | # 24 |

you can do this.

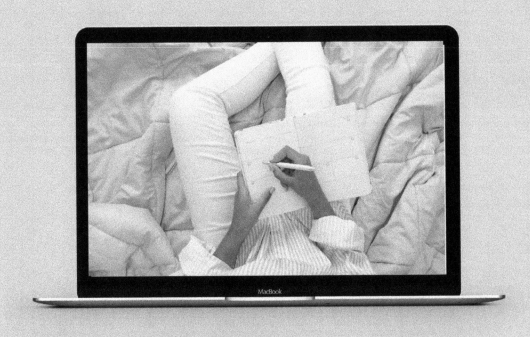

THINKING
AHEAD

● ● ●

A SECTION TO PREPARE YOURSELF FOR
WHAT LIFE THROWS AT YOU

thinking ahead roadMap

QUICK REFERENCE PAGE &
TABLE OF CONTENTS

"YOU LEAVE OLD
HABITS BEHIND
BY STARTING
OUT WITH THE
THOUGHT,
'I RELEASE THE
NEED FOR THIS
IN MY LIFE'"

- WAYNE W. DYER

break the patterns

• • •

24 TIPS TO BREAK OUT OF
TOXIC RELATIONSHIP PATTERNS

24 Tips to Break Your Toxic Patterns

Refer to this page whenever you feel yourself falling into old patterns

TIP 1
Be gentle with yourself.

TIP 2
Practice positive self-talk.

TIP 3
Learn how to be okay with yourself.

TIP 4
Practice setting boundaries.

TIP 5
Stop trying to fix, control, or save.

TIP 6
Find a counselor and consider seeing a psychiatrist for underlying issues (i.e. depression).

TIP 7
Start paying attention to how you talk to yourself.

TIP 8
Find hobbies and things that make you happy on your own.

TIP 9
Practice positive self-talk & tuning out your negative internal voice.

TIP 10
Stop trying to change others.

TIP 11
Accept help from your support system and friends.

TIP 12
Work through your past & childhood wounds.

TIP 13
Learn how to say no to people.

TIP 14
Practice naming your emotions and feelings.

TIP 15
Pay attention to how your body feels.

TIP 16
Read books to help you understand your issues better.

TIP 17
Fully acknowledge you have a pattern of being in toxic relationships.

TIP 18
Focus on living in the present.

TIP 19
Do no contact with your ex.

TIP 20
Give yourself time to heal. Do not date until you are healed.

TIP 21
Explore what relationships were modeled to you as a child.

TIP 22
Assess what your boundaries are.

TIP 23
Do all activities in this workbook.

TIP 24
Accept reality and abandon the fantasy.

you can do this.

"AS SOON AS
YOU TRUST
YOURSELF,
YOU WILL
KNOW HOW
TO LIVE."

-JOHANN WOLFGANG VON
GOETHE, FAUST, FIRST PART

check-in

questions

● ● ●

FOR WHEN YOU START DATING AGAIN

Questions to Ask Yourself

WHEN YOU START DATING AGAIN

Keep these handy and be honest in your answers. If something feels off in the relationship, do not be afraid to walk away and end it.

1

QUESTION

Does this person add value to my life?

2

QUESTION

If this relationship starts going downhill, can I walk away?

3

QUESTION

Am I happy around this person?

4

QUESTION

Do I like this person?

5

QUESTION

Am I attracted to this person?

6

QUESTION

Am I comfortable being myself around this person?

7

QUESTION

Does this relationship give me energy or drain me?

8

QUESTION

Does this person respect me?

9

QUESTION

Have I ever felt unsafe in this relationship?

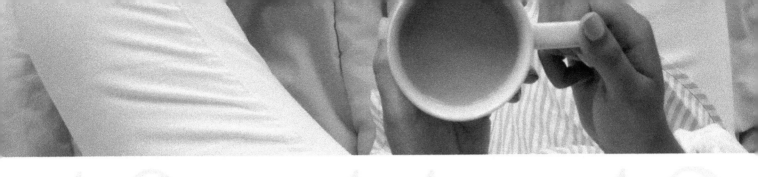

10

QUESTION

Has this person ever made me feel crazy?

11

QUESTION

Has this person violated any of my boundaries?

12

QUESTION

Has this person lied to me?

13

QUESTION

Does this person care about me as a human being?

14

QUESTION

Could I count on this person if I needed something?

15

QUESTION

What's missing from this relationship?

16

QUESTION

Why am I in this relationship?

17

QUESTION

Why am I afraid to end the relationship?

18

QUESTION

Assuming this person never changes, would I be in happy in this relationship?

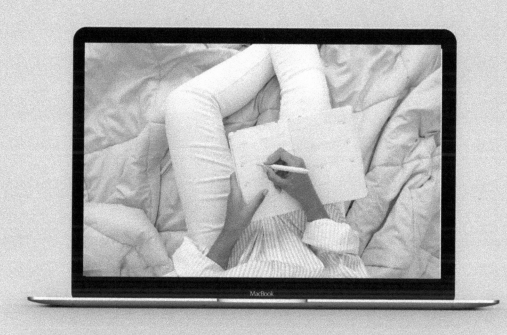

RESOURCES

• • •

FOR WHEN YOU STILL NEED HELP

"BE PATIENT WITH
YOURSELF. SELF-
GROWTH IS TENDER;
IT'S HOLY GROUND.
THERE'S NO GREATER
INVESTMENT."

-STEPHEN COVEY, THE 7 HABITS
OF HIGHLY EFFECTIVE PEOPLE:
POWERFUL LESSONS IN PERSONAL
CHANGE

*top reads &
workbooks*

• • •

MY BOOK & WORKBOOK RECOMMENDATIONS
FOR ALL THE WARRIORS

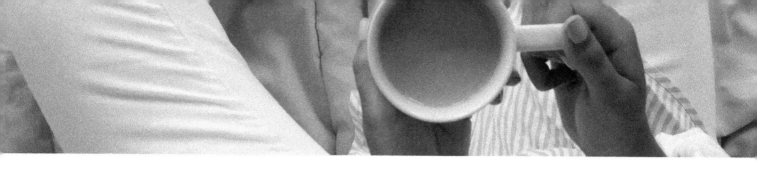

1

BOOK

*Codependent No More:
How to Stop
Controlling Others
and Start Caring
for Yourself
by Melody Beattie*

2

BOOK

*Why Does He Do
That? Inside the
Minds of Angry &
Controlling Men
by Lundy Bancroft*

3

BOOK

*Complex PTSD: From
Surviving to Thriving:
A Guide and Map for
Recovering from
Childhood Trauma
by Pete Walker*

4

BOOK

*The Body Keeps the
Score: Brain, Mind,
and Body in the
Healing of Trauma
by Bessel van der Kolk
M.D.*

5

BOOK

*I Thought It Was Just
Me (but it isn't): Making
the Journey from "What
Will People Think?" to
"I Am Enough"
by Brené Brown, Ph.D.*

6

BOOK

*Why Won't You
Apologize? Healing
Big Betrayals and
Everyday Hurts by
Harriet Lerner, Ph.D*

7

BOOK

*Rage Becomes Her:
The Power of
Women's Anger
by Soraya Chemaly*

8

BOOK

*The Purity Myth:
How America's
Obsession with
Virginity is Hurting
Young Women
by Jessica Valenti*

9

BOOK

*Unspeakable Things:
Sex, Lies, and
Revolution by Laurie
Penny*

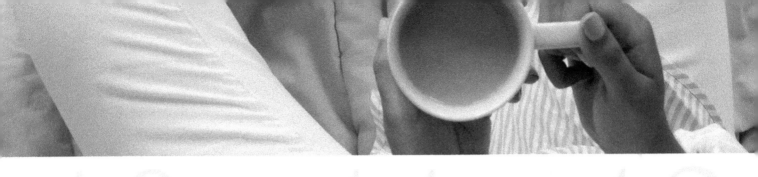

BOOK

The Seven Principles for Making Marriage Work: A Practical Guide from the Country's Foremost Relationship Expert By John M. Gottman, Ph.D. and Nan Silver

BOOK

Nobody's Victim: Fighting Psychos, Stalkers, Pervs, and Trolls by Carrie Goldberg

BOOK

Facing Codependence by Pia Mellody

BOOK

Hold Me Tight: Seven Conversations for a Lifetime of Love by Dr. Sue Johnson

BOOK

The 5 Love Languages: The Secret to Love that Lasts by Gary Chapman

BOOK

The Dance of Anger: A Woman's Guide to Changing the Patterns of Intimate Relationships by Harriet Lerner, Ph.D

BOOK

Untamed by Glennon Doyle

WORKBOOK

The Dialectical Behavior Therapy Skills Workbook by by Matthew McKay PhD, Jeffrey C. Wood PsyD, Jeffrey Brantley MD

WORKBOOK

The Self Esteem Workbook by Glenn R. Schiarldi, Ph.D.

"YOU LOOK AT ME
AND CRY:
EVERYTHING HURTS.
I HOLD YOU AND
WHISPER: BUT
EVERYTHING CAN
HEAL."

- RUPI KAUR

resources

● ● ●

FOR ALL THE WARRIORS

Are you still struggling,

AND YOU WANT TO CONTINUE TO WORK
ON YOUR ISSUES?

Check out these resources.

1

RESOURCE

*Follow
@codependentrecovery
on Instagram for more
tips*

2

RESOURCE

Check out my website

*https://msha.ke/codepen
dentrecovery/*

3

RESOURCE

*Affordable Therapy:
Open Path
Psychotherapy Collective*

openpathcollective.org

4

RESOURCE

*For help if you are
feeling suicidal or in
distress*

*The Lifeline
1-800-273-8255
suicidepreventionlifeline.org*

5

RESOURCE

LGBT Help Center

*National Hotline:
1-888-843-4564*

*Youth Talkline:
1-800-246-7743*

www.glbthotline.org

6

RESOURCE

Crisis Text Line

*Text "HELLO" to
741741*

7

RESOURCE

*Help paying for your
medication*

www.needymeds.org

8

RESOURCE

*National directory of
mental health providers
(US)*

*www.psychologytoday.co
m/us/therapists*

9

RESOURCE

*Co-Dependents
Anonymous: find
support groups*

https://coda.org/

"BABY YOU ARE THE
STRONGEST FLOWER
THAT EVER GREW,
REMEMBER THAT
WHEN THE WEATHER
CHANGES."

-CLEO WADE

resources

• ● •

FOR ALL THE BADASS SURVIVORS

If you are a survivor,
THESE RESOURCES MAY HELP YOU!

This includes resources for domestic violence, sexual assault, revenge porn, campus assault, sex trafficking, stalking, online harassment, and resources geared toward specific populations.

1

RESOURCE

Follow @codependentrecovery on Instagram for more tips

2

RESOURCE

Check out my website

https://msha.ke/codependentrecovery/

3

RESOURCE

National Domestic Violence Hotline

Available 24/7 for chat & calls for women, men, and LGBTQ survivors of domestic violence. They also offer safety planning.

www.thehotline.org
1-800-787-3224

4

RESOURCE

Find a local domestic violence shelter

www.domesticshelters.org

5

RESOURCE

Find free or low cost legal services

www.womenslaw.org/find-help/finding-lawyer

6

RESOURCE

Dating violence laws by state (US)

www.womenslaw.org/laws/general

7

RESOURCE

Information for undocumented victims of domestic violence

www.domesticshelters.org/articles/legal/protection-for-undocumented-victims-of-abuse

8

RESOURCE

Financial tips for leaving

www.moneygeek.com/financial-planning/resources/financial-help-women-abusive-relationships/

9

RESOURCE

How to document abuse

www.loveisrespect.org/pdf/Documenting_Abuse.pdf

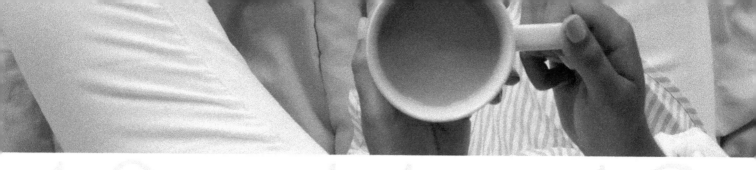

RESOURCE

Creating a safety plan

www.safehorizon.org/our-services/safety-plan/

RESOURCE

For help with COVID-19 approved safety planning

www.sanctuaryforfamilies.org/safety-planning-covid19/

RESOURCE

Domestic violence organizations (US)

www.thehotline.org/resources/victims-and-survivors/

RESOURCE

International survivors

https://hotpeachpages.net/

RESOURCE

Supports youth and young adults in ending dating violence. The website includes planning resources, legal help, educator toolkits, and more

1-800-331-9474
Text: "loveis" to 22522
www.loveisrespect.org

RESOURCE

RAINN (Sexual Assault Survivors)

Available 24/7 for chats & calls [1-800-656-4673].

www.rainn.org

RESOURCE

1IN6 (male sex assault survivors)

Available 24/7 chat Also offers support group meetings

1in6.org

RESOURCE

Stronghearts Native Helpline (American Indian & Alaskan Native survivors)

7 a.m. to 10 p.m. CT.
1-844-762-8483

www.strongheartshelpline.org

RESOURCE

NW Network (LGBTQ survivors)

1-206-568-7777

www.nwnetwork.org

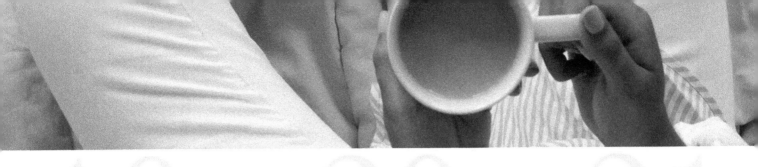

RESOURCE

Crash Override Network: victims of online attacks

crashoverridenetwork. com

RESOURCE

Trans Lifeline (crisis hotline for transgender survivors)

1-877-565-8860
translifeline.org

RESOURCE

National Human Trafficking Hotline

1-888-373-7888

humantraffickinghotli ne.org

RESOURCE

Know Your IX: campus sexual violence or harassment

www.knowyourix.org

RESOURCE

Victims of online harassment

https://iheartmob.org/

RESOURCE

Help getting sexual images or videos down that were posted of you

www.cybercivilrights.org /online-removal/

RESOURCE

CCRI Crisis Helpline (Hotline for victims of nonconsensual pornography)

1-844-878-2274

www.cybercivilrights.org/cc ri-crisis-helpline/

RESOURCE

DMCA Defender (help victims of revenge porn by preventing unauthorized sharing of your images by assisting with DMCA Takedown Notices)

www.dmcadefender.com

RESOURCE

The Stalking Resource Center (helping victims of stalking)

1-202-467-8700

victimsofcrime.org/sta lking-resource-center/